WHY AM I STILL ALIVE?

Surviving Advanced Stage IV Cancer

Yvonne Marie Pigeon

ISBN: 978-1-957453-00-2 (Paperback)
ISBN: 978-1-957453-01-9 (E-book)
Library of Congress Control Number: 2021925879

Big Woods Publications
Green Bay, Wisconsin

www.BigWoodsPublications1.wordpress.com

Front cover image by National Cancer Institute.

Printed in the United States of America.

PREFACE

When Yvonne was first diagnosed, at the age of 53, with advanced stage IV adenocarcinoma, which had metastasized throughout her body, she did not know there might come a day when she would want to write about her experiences — of being misdiagnosed, or being told she probably had six months to live, of undergoing four years of chemotherapy and the endless scans and transfusions, or of the often-surreal feeling of having to live within the confines of a day-to-day struggle simply to endure, and perhaps one day survive.

But survive she did. And because the journey was not an easy one, she came to feel that it might be helpful to tell her story for the benefit of others facing similar circumstances, that they might find reason to hope they too could endure the challenges encountered on the road to recovery. For Yvonne believed that fighting cancer was more than an individual battle — that it was, and continues to be, undertaken by many others at your side as well. So, this medical memoir came to be written.

Yvonne not only survived, but managed to live a long, eventful life, passing away at the age of 80, having become in her remaining years an inspiring example of how giving up should never become an option.

— John Richard Pigeon

I

My arm was bothering me. That's how I remember it starting. I had a sore upper right arm and underarm, which I could not account for. I had not been doing anything out of the ordinary, at least nothing I could think of. Could I have pulled a muscle? Was bursitis setting in? After a week of such thoughts, I went to see my family physician. He examined me, moved my arm this way and that, palpitated it, asked questions, finally coming to the conclusion that there was nothing wrong and that I should try to take it easy for a while and rest the arm as much as possible — and to try to get more sleep.

This advice did not seem to help much. The pain, which grew in intensity as time went on, would not be denied. Soon I was unable to lie on my right side in bed. I decided to return to the doctor. Again, he found nothing out of the ordinary. "Do you sleep near an air conditioner?" he asked. Yes, I did. "Well, that might be your problem. Cold air blowing on a body part can irritate it. I suggest you move your bed away from the rushing air."

I returned home feeling rather foolish. However, the new advice did not seem to help either. The pain in my arm grew so intense after a while that I could hardly function anymore, at work or at home. At night I could lie only on my back, while placing my sore arm on pillows to cushion it. Any pressure at all now on the limb brought nothing short of agony. I paid the doctor a third visit. This time he had his partner examine me. He, too, found nothing out of the ordinary. The X-rays of my arm looked good. So, I was sent home again. By now I was certain the doctors had marked me down as a hypochondriac.

Eventually, I could no longer use my arm to do even everyday things like cooking, or lifting light objects. I couldn't even raise the arm over my head. I called my family physician a fourth time and asked him to recommend a specialist. I was hoping to angle him into doing a biopsy, maybe some kind of exploratory surgery. My family doctor referred me to a surgeon whose opinion was that a stretched pectoral muscle leading into my shoulder area was causing the discomfort, perhaps due to a strain, and would need time to heal. I asked him if he would be doing a biopsy. He looked incredulous and said that he could lose his license if he were to biopsy healthy tissue. I left his office that day walking on air. I finally had a reason for my pain. It wasn't in my head after all. I had a stretched pectoral muscle. I was elated.

Unfortunately, the pain only continued to worsen with time. After a fifth call to my doctor's office, he told me that I had left him with no alternative but to order a bone scan. Fine with me, I thought. Anything to get at the cause of this misery.

During the several weeks all this was going on, and for some time before that actually, I had noticed I was gaining weight—almost twenty-five pounds—and was feeling more fatigued. I was employed at a group home for boys, and although there was some physical labor involved, such as doing laundry and cooking meals, none of these duties had left me feeling fatigued before. Lately, however, something had changed. I remember coming home after work and falling into the recliner for a nap before dinner. As the weeks passed, I found it more difficult to get up from my chair once I was in it. I began to suggest going out for dinner, or picking something up. But that soon got old for all of us. I had mentioned the increased fatigue to my doctor during my first visit, which was the reason he had suggested I try to get more sleep at night. Being a life-long insomniac, I held out little hope for improvement in that area.

The bone scan was scheduled for the following Monday at St. Vincent Hospital in Green Bay. It seemed an easy enough procedure. All I had to do was lie there and listen to the machine make its odd noises, which I remember thinking would bother anyone who had to listen to them all day long. But the technician did not seem bothered at all by the series of nearly-constant beeps the machine was making. In fact, he could not have been a more pleasant and concerned care-giver. I would find out only later what the machine's little beeps meant and perhaps why this very accommodating technician may have felt the need for being so kind to me that morning.

I went to work at the group home the next day as usual and was preparing lunch that noon when my husband, Dick, suddenly showed up at the door. He never was much good at hiding things and I could tell just by looking at him that he had come to tell me something that was going to be difficult for him. He asked if we could speak alone and so I led him into the office where we both sat down. He told me that the doctor had called with the scan results and that they had found a little cancer. I asked him, what did a little cancer mean? But he only said that it would be better if I called the doctor and let him explain things to me. Feeling a bit numbed, I said goodbye to my fellow employees and left with my husband for home. It would be my last day at the group home.

As soon as we got in the door of our house, I phoned and asked to speak with the doctor who had called. In what seems now like a wholly unreal moment, I listened as he told me in the most bluntly dispassionate manner imaginable: "You are loaded with cancer—your vertebrae, your ribs, your pelvis, your leg—it's everywhere." As I sat listening to this man speak with the manner of someone ordering takeout food, I looked over at my husband who had covered his face and was sobbing. So were two of my adult daughters who had come over to the house. They knew what I was hearing.

The doctor continued: "I have notified both the hospital and the oncology department that you will be checking in today. Whoever is on call after office hours in oncology will stop in to see you."

I hung up the phone and rose slowly to my feet. For a moment I wasn't sure I was going to be able to stand up at all. But I did. Dick walked over to me and we hugged and cried without saying anything for a long time. What can anybody say in the face of a death sentence? I was fifty-three years old and I was going to die.

II

I don't remember the ride to the hospital, or checking in, or much of anything else until Dr. McGovern, the assigned oncologist, and his nurse came into the room to speak with me. As I listened, it seemed as if he were talking about someone else. I had to continually remind myself that all of this was occurring to *me.*

Then, as soon as he had come, he was gone and I was left to the realization that I had to start thinking differently if I was to comprehend what was happening. It still seemed so surreal. That morning I had woken up as the presumably healthy mother of six grown children, had gone to work as usual, and had planned to come home to make meatloaf and scalloped potatoes that evening for supper. Instead, I was now lying in a hospital bed, my family surrounding me in tears. Was it really all over? Was I to remain in this hospital room to the end? No way. I had birthday presents to buy, Christmas shopping to do, grandchildren to spoil. I wasn't *ready* to go yet. Later, my youngest son and his wife informed me that they had found out they were expecting their second child on the very day I went into the hospital, but didn't want to mention it that night because they didn't know my prognosis. Would I still be alive for the birth of their baby?

After a while I told my family to go home until we knew more. In truth, I couldn't bear to look at their hopelessly sad faces any longer. I also told my husband to go back to the house and try to get some rest. It was going to be a long haul from now on and we would both need all the strength we could muster. But he knew that the doctor was coming back later to question me further and he wanted to be there. I couldn't blame him for wanting to stay.

At about seven o'clock that evening Dr. McGovern returned without his nurse to give me a preliminary examination. By this time, two of my cousins, both registered nurses, had come to the hospital. Dr. McGovern said that he had many questions he needed to ask me and did I want my visitors to leave the room. I told him they could stay. He nodded and immediately began to pepper me with questions non-stop for almost an hour. When he was finished gathering all the information he needed, he closed his notebook and said that he wanted to make two things clear. "First, if your treatment here does not show signs of success," he said, "I will recommend you to Johns Hopkins in Baltimore. However, you need to be aware that, as a world-famous facility, it would be expensive." That's all right, I muttered, we wouldn't have the funds for that anyway. "Secondly," he went on, "I won't let you suffer if it comes to that." My puzzled look led to his explanation. "In England," he said, "physicians are allowed to administer medical doses of heroine, which allow the patient to remain coherent enough to communicate with loved ones right up to the end. But here in the U.S., heroine for medical treatment is outlawed. We would have to place you on morphine. The downside of morphine is that it dopes the patient up to the point where they are, in the final days, in a comatose-like state, which naturally would not allow for much communication with loved ones. On the positive side, you would not be in pain."

Both of my RN cousins told me afterwards, as did Dick, how impressed they were with the thoroughness of Dr. McGovern's interview with me. So was I.

Soon after the doctor left, my three well-wishers said goodbye for the night. It was nearly eight o'clock and visiting hours were pretty much over with anyway. Now that I was alone, I began to think about things until I couldn't stand it any longer. I had to get up, maybe walk around some. My room was at the end of a long hall, so I decided to cover the distance of the corridor and back. I was on the ninth floor, which was reserved for cancer patients, so there were many other very ill people around. I walked slowly (where was I going to go, after all?), past the doorways of other patients, past the nurses' station, continuing down the hall. The stillness of the place seemed both comforting and yet disconcerting at the same time. I was almost to the end of the corridor when I noticed a woman standing in the doorway of one of the rooms. I looked at her; she smiled. And then something happened that has never happened to me before or since. The woman held out her arms as if she would hug me. I was so filled with grief and despair I stopped walking and we held each other. It was so spontaneous. I sobbed on her shoulder, "I don't want to have cancer." She patted me gently on the back. We stood that way without speaking for a time and then I thanked her and turned to head back to my room. I don't know if she was a patient, a staff member, or perhaps just a kind visitor. During the two weeks I was in the hospital, I never met up with her again. That night I slept without dreaming.

III

St. Vincent Hospital at that time had three oncologists with offices in the building, and I got to know all three after a while. Although friends suggested I seek treatment at a more well-known medical center, such as the Mayo Clinic or some other prestigious place, I felt very confident that I was in good hands and saw no reason to go elsewhere. In the end, it would turn out to be a fortunate choice. Having first been seen by Dr. McGovern, and having liked him, I retained him as my primary oncologist.

Since the X-rays revealed that I had a great deal of cancerous lesions along the surfaces of my bones, Dr. McGovern had to explain to me that bone cancer of this nature was always secondary. Therefore, it was going to be necessary to locate the source. In females, he said, the disease usually begins in the ovaries or in the breast tissue before metastasizing or spreading to the bones. He told me that I had a heavy concentration of tumors along my ribs and vertebrae, as well as my pelvis and left femur. His plan was to call in an orthopedic specialist to biopsy my pelvic area and another surgeon to do a biopsy of the tissue on the right side of my upper torso. There were also more tests, X-rays, and scans to be done. The scans were the worst, because for some of them my arms had to be held above my head for the pictures to turn out. My right arm from the shoulder to the elbow was still as painful as ever and I could not hold back my annoying tears while having to extend my arms like that for the duration of the procedure.

However, the scans did prove valuable in identifying an area of shading under my right arm, along the chest wall. This area, Dr. McGovern said, would have to be biopsied. When the surgeon who performed the tissue extraction (the same fellow who had told me two weeks earlier that I had a stretched pectoral muscle) came to visit me afterwards, he said that there was cancer wherever he looked, in every direction. “We definitely found the mother lode,” was how he phrased it. He spoke as if he were talking about a vein of precious metal. The pelvic biopsy also revealed a solid concentration of tumors.

I don’t recall how many days it took before all of the tests were completed, but when they were, Dr. McGovern came into my room to speak with Dick and me. He was a man of average height with an easy manner and a steady eye who took his job very seriously, even while managing to demonstrate true compassion, a trait the biopsy surgeon could have used more of. Dr. McGovern explained that there were five stages of cancer, the fifth stage being death. He told me that I had an advanced stage IV adenocarcinoma. The originating tumor, which he described as being shaped like a large, elongated pancake, had embedded itself in my ribs and spinal column in such a way that surgery was no longer an option. He added that judging by its size and the extent to which it had metastasized, the tumor had probably been growing for about two years, having now spread to nearly every part of my body by means of my skeletal system. I asked him how long he thought I had. He said that was a question no one could answer, that there was just no way of knowing. I told him I appreciated his forthrightness in any case, as I had things I needed to get in-order first. He remained to talk with us at length, answering all of our questions as if he had nothing else to do in the world, despite the late hour. I then asked if there were any options at all. "Oh definitely," he answered. Although I was not a candidate for radiation, since the cancer was so pervasive, he told me I *was* an ideal candidate for chemotherapy, and that treatment would begin immediately. "We aren't giving up," he said. "We're going to attack this malignancy." A final comment, made in passing, was how fortunate it was that no major organs were involved yet. After he left, Dick and I just looked at each other. It was all so dreadful to think about that neither of us could think of anything to say.

IV

Eventually I was fitted with a catheter, called a Hickman, inserted into the center of my chest so that the chemotherapy (chemical therapy) could be administered directly. This device was deemed necessary as the veins in my arm were neither large enough nor easy enough to find in order to support regular injections. The thing about chemotherapy, Dr. McGovern had explained, was that these powerful drugs, although effective on cancer cells, killed indiscriminately, destroying many healthy cells as well. My blood would have to be monitored regularly to make sure the cell count was not being depleted too quickly. Blood transfusions would be needed whenever this occurred. "I'm putting you on the strongest stuff available," he said. "A combination designed to work against your particular type of cancer. It will wreak havoc with your body but it will kill the cancer cells as well. You will lose your hair; you will feel fatigued; you may well lose your appetite; you may even feel nausea at the very idea of food. But you must try to eat, even if you don't feel like it, as caloric intake is the only way to keep your strength up in the fight ahead."

Well, the good doctor certainly knew what

he was talking about. Within weeks of my first chemotherapy treatment, I was as bald as an egg. Even my eyebrows fell out. Every morning after my first few treatments I would wake up to a handful of hair on my pillow before heading for the bathroom to wash up. I remember standing in front of the mirror, looking at myself. It was clear that I was staring at the reflection of a very ill person. And that person was me. I looked terrible.

By the time I returned to my bed, one of my daughters, who helped a lot in those early days, would have removed the clumps of hair and cleaned up as best she could in so short a time. She told me months later that she had hoped to spare me that "sick bed" sight. But I had already seen it for myself earlier.

The fatigue I began to feel had me sleeping for up to twenty hours a day during the first few weeks. But the doctor was, happily, wrong on one account: my appetite never lagged, nor did I suffer much nausea. In fact, after receiving my treatments, usually early in the morning, Dick and I would often go out for breakfast. When I mentioned this to Dr. McGovern, he seemed surprised but pleased for me. "That's wonderful," he enthused. "Let's hope it continues." Later on, he told me that my cast-iron stomach, as he called it, was one of the reasons for my ability to stay on chemo for so long. He also informed me about this time that the reason for the original symptomatic pain in my right arm was probably due to the pressure the tumor had exerted on a nerve leading from my spine into my arm. At least that mystery was solved.

I received chemotherapy injections every four weeks at the oncology office in the hospital. At the time, all chemotherapy drugs at St. Vincent's were kept in bins of chipped ice and were mixed by nurses into individual chemical "cocktails" for each patient according to their oncologist's orders. The chemo effects, mainly a fatigue bordering on exhaustion in my case, would last about two weeks, after which I would feel fairly okay for the remaining two weeks before it was time for more injections. Then the monthly cycle would begin again. Dick, who acted as my nurse at home, kept my Hickman catheter clean with Heparin rinses, via injection, which he had been instructed to administer by the nurses. Since catheter sites sometimes had the tendency to become infected, it was necessary to keep the area around them thoroughly and regularly cleaned and dried. I could not shower because of the chest tube, and instead had to take what I called birdbaths. I have to say that Dick was very diligent about it all, doing his nursing chores and administering my other medications with neither complaints nor dereliction of duty. Other members of the family did their best to help as well. My eldest son, who immediately went out to research alternative treatments for my disease, discovered something called macrobiotics, a method of supposedly purifying the body of carcinogens while building the immune system through a radical change of diet. Trouble was that the diet, made up mostly of whole grains, seemed to me more fitting for a domestic farm animal than a human who was used to meat and potatoes. I remember my husband's droll description of the diet as "tying on the feedbag" providing for one of the few moments of mirth during those intense early days.

One of my daughters offered to make our meals using the macrobiotic cookbook, and for a month or so we did give it a try. But in the end, we were simply not able to stick to it. I just couldn't face another plate of food that looked as if it had already been chewed. I can still recall our last macro meal: a plate of seaweed and beans. As we ate, tears began to flow down my cheeks, until eventually we all started laughing at our pathetic efforts at simply trying to swallow the stuff. Finally, it was decided that we would cut as much red meat from our diet as possible, eat more fruits and vegetables, and just let nature take its course regarding diet.

Another daughter of ours—we have four, along with two sons—offered to come regularly to clean the house, which was also very much appreciated. One son-in-law had rigged up a special bed in the living room so that I would not have to be confined to my bedroom in back, as I was still spending about twenty hours a day dozing on and off.

But while all of these generous and loving efforts helped, things were certainly not easy. And as smoothly as the day-to-day treatment of my condition appeared to be running, we all knew it might be just a matter of time before the end.

V

I have to be honest here and say that I actually cannot recall much about those first two months at home and have had to rely on hospital records and doctor's notes in preparing this memoir. I've also had to rely on the memories of those closest to me during that dark period of my life. When I did read the records and notes and heard what my family had to say of those days, I was taken aback. According to Doctor McGovern's notes, I was "experiencing severe depression, agitation, crying episodes, in addition to a marked fatigue due to the effects of her chemotherapy." The fatigue I remember. But that's about all. I asked Dick if he thought the doctor might have exaggerated in the notes, and he answered, "Not really," before adding, "it's not that you were moping around and moaning 'why me?' all the time. It's just that you were sad, very sad—and frightened—at the idea that you probably didn't have very long to live. You simply weren't ready to die yet; that's what you kept saying." An entry from the journal of one of my daughters addresses those difficult times:

> I went there to cook supper tonight and she was very tired. I made cod, baked potatoes, and green beans, all favorites of hers. She

> hardly ate any of it, she was so down. Dad, out of frustration, told me, "You're going to have to start making something she can eat." I don't know what to do. In some ways his life has been just as upset as hers has by all of this.

According to Dr. McGovern's notes, I was placed on Desyrel, an anti-depressant. The notes also mention that I did not tolerate very well the narcotic analgesic Percocet, prescribed for pain, and so was switched to Motrin 800mg and Tylenol #3. But all of this, too, is a blur to me. When I wasn't sleeping, I was apparently lost in a haze of fear and dejection. Certainly not a pretty picture to be caught up in. For several weeks I had done very little but doze, eat, cry, and take my medications before falling back into a fitful sleep. Such were the effects on the body, I was told, of the poisons being pumped regularly into my system to combat the carcinoma that had come to dinner and decided to stay.

Part of the adverse effects were low blood counts, called "pancytopenia," which I began to experience within a month of first taking chemotherapy. By then I had started emerging from my mind-fog long enough to become coherent and even sociable. As I had always enjoyed playing multi-card bingo at the local casino, my daughter thought I might benefit from a night out for a change, and decided to take me there. But we had no sooner sat down at our table when my body suddenly began to shake all over. At first, I thought I might just be chilled, but the shaking wouldn't stop. In fact, it quickly grew worse. I wasn't just shivering, I was *shaking* badly, as if suffering from advanced Parkinson's. My daughter, seeing the condition I was in, asked someone to call for an ambulance, which soon arrived.

Once at the hospital, I learned my blood count levels had become so low that I could well have died that night. The next day, after I'd undergone a transfusion, Dr. McGovern told me I was lucky to still be among the living, and that we'd have to start monitoring my blood more often from then on. There were times during my treatment when my white blood cell count dropped to as low as 1.9 (a healthy person's count is around 7.0), my red blood cell count to as low as 1.7 (rather than the 4.0 of a healthy person), and my platelet count to as low as 56, which is quite a bit below the normal level of 230. The situation at the hospital that night had been so critical, I learned, that several of my children had begun preparations for coping with what they thought might be my last night alive.

Another of the Doctor's notes mentions that I had called his office one day, saying I could really use some peer support, which led to my attending a cancer-patient group. However, as much as I very much continue to encourage others to seek out such groups, I quickly discovered that I was not going to be an exemplary member of any of them. In my case, it seemed absurd to sit there listening to the cheerful optimism of a woman who'd undergone a lumpectomy. And when I *did* meet up with someone who was indeed very sick, I didn't know what to say to her. I remember one patient at the meeting, a lovely young woman with long blonde hair who must have been in her twenties. Her face was as grey as ash, her beautiful blue eyes already beginning to look sunken. Within months she was dead.

Another woman, about thirty years old, said she had two small children at home. It was quite clear that she was losing whatever battle she was fighting and would soon be leaving her two children behind. I could hardly stand the thought of it. What could I possibly say to these women? There I was with a stage IV carcinoma eating me up from the inside out and yet I looked healthier than they did, healthier than many of them.

Over the course of my treatment, I saw the

faces of many oncology patients come and go, some young, some not so young. After a while I stopped asking the nurses where so-and-so was today, because all too often the answer was that he or she had passed away last month, or last week, or yesterday. I don't know how anyone can work in the field of oncology, with patient mortality rates so high. They are special people indeed.

I remember asking Dr. McGovern once, "What *is* cancer, anyway? Where does it come from?" His answer managed to both fascinate and frighten me. He explained that cancer was, put simply, the uncontrolled dividing of cells. Somehow the mechanism for replication becomes defective, as if it were stuck in the "on" position, so to speak, and that it was the job of oncologists to one day find a way to switch it off again, if possible. As to what *caused* the disease, he said there was still much to be learned about that part of it. While it seemed obvious that overexposure to the sun played a factor in melanoma, and that tobacco was a factor in lung and oral cancers, the triggers for many malignancies were still shrouded in mystery. And often there appeared to be no rhyme or reason to it. Why, for instance, could some people smoke heavily for fifty years and not develop lung cancer, while others, who never lit up a cigarette in their lives, succumb to the disease?

So, I shied away from the cancer support groups, disregarded the philosophical enigmas of the disease, and tried to take things one day at a time, to deal with each new development only as it came up. If I needed a transfusion, then I got one. If my catheter site became infected, then I took the antibiotics necessary to clear it up. That's how you get through it, dealing with one thing at a time, as it arises. *And* by not thinking too long or hard about any of it. The existential dread of contemplating one's own impending death can be terrifying — and a good waste of time and energy. Fortunately, as the weeks and months passed, such depressing thoughts occurred less and less frequently, and usually only late at night when I had trouble falling asleep.

I remember one particularly restless night lying in bed listening to a national nighttime radio show. It was the open-phones segment of the program, so I decided to call in. I didn't really think I'd get on, but I figured what the heck, it was one more way of killing time until daylight. When, to my surprise, I was suddenly connected to the host, I couldn't think of anything to say. So, I just told him how grateful I was to have someone to listen to during the long night. I wanted him to know the comfort he had brought to a cancer patient. He asked me what kind of cancer I had and what my situation was. I explained that I had terminal breast cancer.

"How do you know for sure that it's terminal?" he asked. I answered that I could only go by what my physicians had communicated to me. I can't remember much else that was said, but after a few kind words of encouragement, he wished me luck and we ended our conversation. After hanging up, I continued to think about the gist of what he'd said, that doctors weren't *infallible*, after all. I wanted so badly to believe in his optimism. Yet I was not one to kid myself, either. I had inside of me a cancer that had somehow spread to every area of my body, with the lone exceptions of my arms and feet. I could not delude myself about that fact. And yet I can't remember ever feeling entirely hopeless either. People were known to have come back from conditions as desperate as mine, although such cases were admittedly rare. Why couldn't I be one of the exceptions? After much consideration, I decided that a guarded optimism was not unreasonable—that a person could prepare for the worst even while striving for something better.

VI

When you're considered terminal, the idea is never far from your mind, even on those days when you don't feel particularly ill, which in my case was about half the days out of each month. And if you sometimes forgot about the severity of your condition, there were always small reminders to bring you back to reality. I can remember sitting in my recliner at home one afternoon watching some silly talk show (the makeshift bed had been removed from the living room by this time). One of our younger grandchildren—she must have been four or five years old—was over and happened to be looking out the bay window when she suddenly saw one of her aunts pull up into the driveway. Excited, she ran to the backdoor to greet the visitor. I could hear the enthusiasm in her voice as she described her day at Grandma's house. Then she took her aunt by the hand and brought her into the living room where I was sitting. The child looked and sounded so cute I couldn't help but smile. Then she pointed to me and said, "Doesn't Grandma look funny in her wig?" Later my daughter told me that my reaction to this blunt yet truthful observation was to simply lay my head back on the headrest and close my eyes, my smile slowly dissolving away.

I can also remember going to lunch one day with my two nurse cousins and my elderly aunt, mother to one of the cousins. This aunt, a very dear woman who had been, during my youth, like a second mother to me, was now in her eighties and showing the telltale symptoms of Alzheimer's disease. As we talked over lunch, my aunt appeared to notice for the first time that I had lost most of my hair. Although she had been told on numerous occasions by her daughter that I had cancer and had lost my hair to chemotherapy, she could not help asking me why I didn't let my hair grow out. Her daughter, perhaps grown frustrated, turned to her and said, "Mother, don't you know that Eve is dying?"

Of course, my cousin had not said anything that those of us sitting there were unaware of, but until then I had never actually heard the words spoken aloud by anyone before and I remember being surprised by the simple finality of the phrase. As matter-of-fact as the words were, I had needed to hear them, and I was grateful to my cousin. Although Dr. McGovern had also communicated this same truth to me, in so many words, not even he had used the word 'dying'. Yet, within the month he would be given the opportunity. It was during my second trip to the hospital for an emergency transfusion due to low blood counts. I was lying in bed, every bit as sick as such a condition will make one feel, when he came into the room. After a brief discussion of this latest complication, I took a breath and asked him pointblank, “Am I dying?” I can still see him standing by the window before a beautiful early morning sky. His voice was soft yet audible. “Yes,” he said. I lifted my hands to my face and started crying. While I wept, I heard the sound of shoes along the floor. Dr. McGovern had walked to the side of the bed. After a moment’s pause, he placed his hand on my shoulder. Such a simple gesture, yet so welcome to one in such misery.

Other than that quiet moment, there was never another mention of the obvious, but rather, if anything, a renewed concentration on combating the disease in whatever manner possible. He knew that even a few more months would mean everything to a dying mother and grandmother. And, my goodness, was he thorough. I can recall once complaining to him about an ongoing headache I’d been experiencing. Nothing seemed to help, I told him. Just a dull continuous ache in the head. Since I had already established myself as a patient who was not a complainer, he decided that a brain scan should be done. By the next morning I was all set to be brought down to X-ray. But as I waited, something bothered me. I'd had this same kind of nuisance headache before, many times. And then it hit me — this was an *allergy* headache. I was sure of it as soon as the thought came to me. It was autumn and my twice-yearly (spring and fall) headaches were returning, as they always did. A panel test done at an allergy clinic once revealed that I was allergic to almost everything that grew, from ragweed to maple trees. I was also told I couldn't eat chocolate, coffee beans, salmon, shellfish, among many other things, without inducing a headache, although I have often put up with the annoyance when it comes to shellfish and salmon, both favorites.

When the nurse came to get me, I explained to her why I was suddenly refusing the scan. "Dr. McGovern won't like this," she said.

"Well, Dr. McGovern will have to understand," I answered.

She warned me, "He's pretty determined when it comes to ruling things out, you know."

"Yes, I know," I said, "and sometimes it can be a real pain in the butt."

"Well, don't let him know about *that* pain," she replied dryly, "God knows what kind of tests he'd order for that." It was this kind of levity that helped as much as anything in the long battle ahead.

As it turned out, Dr. McGovern did understand, and so, however reluctantly, canceled the order for the brain scan. I was impressed by the fact that he did not feel the need to overrule my own experience in this matter. But then, power issues were never a problem with him. He knew what needed to be done and when, as well as what might *not* need to be done at a particular time. Besides, we were both well aware that my quarterly body scan was coming up in a few weeks, so I'm sure he figured he still had all the bases covered anyway, despite me and my expertise.

VII

I saw the doctor every week at first, then every other week for a while. I continued to have troubles with blood count levels and was still feeling zapped of strength for those first few weeks after each chemotherapy session. I remember when one of my daughters came over to make a kettle of vegetable soup for lunch. It was so delicious I ended up eating two bowls. I am not one of the fortunate few who eat to live, but rather one of those who too often live to eat. In any case, early that same afternoon I had an appointment with Dr. McGovern. Blood tests done there indicated I was seriously low on platelets and would need to check into the hospital immediately for a transfusion. I suppose I'd been caught on a bad day, but I simply did not want to go back into the hospital again. So, I refused. In fact, I exited the office and walked out to the waiting room like a defiant child. I didn't care. I was just so sick of being sick.

Dr. McGovern waited a moment before walking out to where I was and sitting down beside me. "Eve," he said (he always called me by my nickname), "nobody likes going back into the hospital, but you really don't have a choice here. Your blood needs to be replenished." Of course, he was right, and of course I would check back into the hospital. I guess I just needed to feel sorry for myself before doing what I knew had to be done. I was in the hospital by three o'clock that afternoon. Although I had experienced regular blood transfusions, I had never received both blood cells and platelets at the same time before.

Wouldn't you know it, as soon as the procedure was over, I immediately began feeling nauseated and very shortly afterwards spewed up all that delicious vegetable soup my daughter had made for lunch. I hurled for hours. Later, Dr. McGovern explained to me that receiving so much blood material at once, especially platelets, often caused such a reaction in patients unused to the process.

In addition to hospital stays for the occasional transfusion, I would once in a while have to check in due to an infection developing around my chest catheter. During these episodes, I would be hooked up to an IV containing antibiotics. Later, on other occasions when the catheter site became infected, I was sent home with the materials necessary to treat the infection myself. During these times, Dick would again act as my nurse, carefully cleaning the catheter site with antibiotic wipes every six hours, after which he would hook me up to an IV drip that took about half an hour to empty, entering via the chest tube. This process had to be repeated every six hours without fail for three days, even through the night. It wasn't difficult, just tiring, especially those midnight drips which seemed to take hours. Yet, once again Dick never complained about having to get up and get everything ready and going.

After a while the office visits were down to once a month, during which time I would have my regular blood work done and receive my usual dose of chemotherapy. Most of these visits became so routine that it's hard to distinguish one from another. But there was one visit I recall quite vividly. I had just entered the hospital when I noticed a man sitting in one of the hallways at a table set up with all kinds of items. I have always loved receiving free samples of things and thought I'd stop by and see what the fellow was offering. Upon reaching the table, though, I learned that he was a salesman from a pharmaceutical company and had come to show the physicians the latest array of new wonder drugs available. After explaining this to me, he said, "So I guess I can't be of much service to you."

"That's all right" I quipped, "I buy all my drugs on the street," and walked away.

Five minutes later I was escorted into Dr. McGovern's office, and the first thing he said to me when he finally came in was, "So, how long have you been buying your drugs on the street?" Turns out he'd been sitting in the doctor's lounge across from the display table and had heard my wry comment to the salesman. I felt a bit foolish at having been overheard, but joined him in a chuckle anyway.

* * *

As I had long ago lost all my hair to the effects of the chemotherapy, I decided that I'd better look into the possibility of buying a wig of my own, having borrowed one of my sister's wigs for long enough. So, I went to a specialty shop and browsed, all the while listening to the saleswoman explain to me that since I would be wearing the wig for a while *and* since I would be older once my hair finally grew back—she had no notion of my rather bleak prognosis—I might want to consider a wig with some grey in it. I had not been grey when I lost my hair, but I was fifty-three years old. I myself had heard somewhere that returning hair is often greyer for people who have undergone chemotherapy. So, although both my mother and grandmother had lived long lives without ever turning grey,

I listened to her when I probably shouldn't have and purchased two wigs, both with a fair amount of grey in them.

I was surprised how *uncomfortable* wigs could be when worn during warm weather. By that summer they had become so uncomfortable that I decided not to wear them at all, with the exception of special occasions such as weddings, formal gatherings, and the like. Instead, I started going around in all my glorious baldness to the store, to cribbage night at the VFW, practically everywhere. I'd given up caring what I looked like, as long as I didn't have to sweat under those ridiculous mops of hair anymore. Interestingly enough, when my hair finally did start growing back, it was neither grey nor my original color — it was pure white. Not only that, but it had lost all of its natural wave and was as straight as fishing line. I could hardly believe it. Fortunately, this change was only temporary, and before long all the stiff white hair fell out and was replaced with hair of my natural color and texture again. Eventually, I ended up throwing the wigs away, which I regret, as I've since learned that donating wigs to oncology departments is both appreciated and encouraged.

After the first few months of depression had passed, my attitude steadily became more positive. I'd always been an optimist and it looked like I was to remain one. Naturally, I was aware that I was still a stage IV cancer patient, but by the following spring I didn't *feel* like one. Although my disease was always in the back of my mind, I never felt the way I had imagined a dying person should feel. This wasn't a case of denial. I just didn't feel all that sick. I was convinced that I had to be getting better. Just a few months later I would learn that these feelings of improvement were not that far off the mark.

VIII

I have in this memoir referred several times to what is called a body or bone scan. Actually, the radiology department's official name for it is "body bone scan." Let me take a moment to explain what actually goes on during one of these procedures, since they are the basic means for keeping track of the metastatic cancer process. I would also add here that scans and tests are always being improved, becoming much more refined and less time-consuming. The following is how I experienced them at the time.

First, I was injected intravenously with a mildly radioactive solution, in my case about 24 mCi of Technetium 99mTc MDP. This then had to circulate for three hours before the scan could be taken, thus allowing time for full absorption, in turn allowing the radiologist to see if there are any new areas of tumor growth or activity going on. He/she would also be able to detect if there is any lessening of activity. So, I always had three hours to kill before the scan could proceed, which Dick and I usually spent in any number of ways, from playing cards to getting something to eat.

After the three-hour waiting period was up, I was brought to the scanning room's large table, on which I was positioned. Pillows were placed under my head and knees for comfort, as it was important that one remained as still as possible during the procedure. Back then, a full-body scan required that the patient lay on his or her back while a large rectangular device was lowered to within inches of the body. This device would then slowly (and I do mean slowly) progress from the area of the head to the feet, scanning first the right side. After it had reached as far as the feet, it would then start moving slowly back again, this time scanning the left side. This two-cycle process was called the 'anterior' scan, and took about forty minutes. I then turned over in order for the 'posterior' scan of both sides of my body to be completed. Today, fortunately, the procedure takes much less time.

It was that first full-body scan that revealed how the cancer had metastasized to nearly every part of my body by traveling along my skeletal system. In the beginning, I underwent a scan every two or three months in order to see how the chemotherapy treatments were affecting the cancer's progression, after which Dr. McGovern would receive the radiology report. Often these reports containing the same line: "There are multiple areas of increased activity noted." Most of the areas of increased tumor activity involved my vertebrae and rib cage, where the massive tumor of origination was still deeply rooted and inoperable. The only good news about the reports was that there appeared to be no new tumors to add to those already present. At least I didn't appear to be getting any worse, which, granted, wasn't saying a whole lot when talking about a stage IV malignancy.

But then, one day, while listening to Dr. McGovern tell me about the results of my latest body scan, I heard him say something I never thought I'd ever hear. He told me the radiology report revealed "improvement in most of the bone lesions." Apparently, the many smaller tumors which had spread along my skeletal system had not only ceased spreading, they were, in Dr. McGovern's words, "in partial remission." I was stunned at hearing the news and asked him if this meant I might have a chance of recovery.

Not wanting to kill the optimism of the moment, yet not wanting to plant unrealistic hopes in my head either, he said I needed to understand that the originating tumor was still unaffected, and in fact continued to show increased activity along my vertebrae and ribs. I told him I understood. And yet, as we spoke, I could tell that even he, cautious as he always was and would remain, could not help being impressed by the unexpected appearance of this "partial remission".

Dr. McGovern's cautiousness was of course the product of having seen so many cancer patients over the years. People simply did not survive my kind of stage IV carcinoma. An overly optimistic approach would have been ill-founded, and in fact a body scan in August once more revealed "multiple areas of increased activity noted through thoracic and lumbar vertebrae with involvement of upper ribs." By the following January the radiologist's impression was:

> Bone scan reveals areas of increased activity through the skeletal system suggestive of metastatic disease with no major interval change when compared with previous study.

So, was I getting better or not? According to a note made by Dr. McGovern in May of that year, "the patient's pain is completely resolved. At this time her malignancy has no evidence of progressive symptomology." In June, he reported, "I can detect no fullness in the axilla of right breast as previously noted." And by August, the first anniversary of my diagnosis, his notes reveal, "Bone scan and chest X-ray show stabilization of her disease with no evidence of progression." If I wasn't getting any better, at least I wasn't getting any worse either.

Thus, even though the main tumor was alive and thriving, I was apparently going to hang around a bit longer than any of us had originally supposed I would. The chemo-therapy, however, was still so devastating to my blood count levels that I continued to need occasional transfusions of both cells and platelets. The effects of these powerful drugs would eventually lead Dr. McGovern to reduce the intensity of chemo treatments until my body could resolve some of its blood issues on its own. After I had recuperated some, he would raise the doses to an intermediate level, in time ordering the levels to be returned to their original dosages.

Around this same time, I was also hospitalized for deep venous thrombophlebitis (blood clot) in my lower leg, which called for the administration of the anti-coagulant drug Coumadin, a medication I would stay on for some time to come, due to my tendency to develop clots.

These small steps, some forward, some backwards, continued throughout the first six months of the second year. Then, in June, came the following radiology report, as revealed in Dr. McGovern's notes:

> There are very few small areas of increased activity through thoracic vertebrae with subtle area of minimally increased activity in right 5th and right 7th ribs with no major interval change when compared with previous study of six months ago. Bone scan reveals evidence of metastatic disease in remission.

In further notes, Dr. McGovern would write simply: "Bone scan shows remission of her disease." By the second anniversary of my diagnosis, he was able to record, "Patient remains in a clinical state of remission. Reduction of chemo again due to low counts."

I *was* getting better.

IX

But stabilization of a disease, I found, was not synonymous with conquering it. I had a ways to go yet before I could begin to consider myself any kind of survivor, although my optimism did receive a boost from the good news. And here is as good a place as any, I suppose, to say that I firmly believe one's *outlook* is absolutely fundamental in the way he or she goes about battling a cancer, or any other disease for that matter. A belief that you can get better is vital. Ever since I was a child I have, like so many people, had to struggle every inch of the way through life. Nothing came easy. But I was fortunate in that I always believed things could, and would, get better. And they usually did. All my life I've felt this way, which may be one of the reasons I'm still around to talk about it. I can even remember telling amusing stories to Dr. McGovern during examinations, which left us both laughing. Humor is contagious. And so is hope, especially in the face of difficulty. In fact, Dr. McGovern once told me that he enjoyed having me as his first patient of the morning as it always left him feeling more upbeat the rest of the day. So, try to find something to smile about. It's helpful, in more ways than one.

Meanwhile, I continued to experience hospitalizations due to the effects of the chemotherapy. (Over the course of my treatment, I would be hospitalized four times for emergency transfusions, five times for DVT or lower legs clots, and five times for chest catheter infections.) But one thing was for certain: the cancer wasn't tolerating the ill effects of the chemo any better than I was. Most importantly, the drug treatments had not affected my ability to eat. I could take in food to replenish my energy levels; I could receive healthy blood products when needed; I could even mow the lawn again, and so was building up strength. I had emotional and physical support on all sides. The cancer had no such resources. And in time it began to show, even on the large, inoperable tumor of origination.

I suppose I don't need to explain that a cancer patient, for various reasons, often has to take medications other than the chemotherapy drugs. A list of the meds I received at different times during treatment would include the following: Toprol 25mg, Aricept 10mg, Diovan 20mg,

Hydrochlorothiazide 25mg, Ambien 10mg, Quinine Sulfate 260mg, Klor-Con 10mg, Warfarin 5mg, Triamterene 75mg, Coumadin 5mg, and Potassium 10mEq. Later I was placed on Tamoxifen 10mg, and after that, Arimidex 1mg daily.

I also found it helpful to remember that some aches and pains are going to be the result not of one's fight against lethal disease but because of the body's natural changes over time, especially if the patient in question is over fifty, as I was. Throughout my ordeal, I had complaints of numerous aches and pains that often turned out upon examination to be only the inevitable deterioration of aging joints and other bodily parts.

In my case the pain was due largely to osteoarthritis, which was gradually affecting different areas of my skeletal system, such as my hips, knees, ankles, shoulders, wrists, hands, and spinal column. Every time I had a flare up of bone pain, I would think that the cancer might once again be advancing. During one visit to Dr. McGovern's office, brought about by one or another of these aches and pains—which of course he had to explore in order to rule out any possible recurrence of cancer, tests of which always turned out negative—I remember him saying to me in good humor, "You, my friend, are F.O.S."

I looked at him and said, "Doctor, I may be full of cancer, but I am not full of sh-t." He laughed out loud, adding, "Oh, I see you're sharper this morning than I thought."

X

In every case history there comes a moment of truth when things will inevitably end up going one way or the other, for better or worse. One can only hope and work toward the better.

In March of my third year of treatment, a day I won't soon forget, Dr. McGovern wrote down the following sentence in his notes about me: "Bone scan today shows complete remission of her disease." I can't begin to explain what hearing that phrase meant to me. I was not going to die of metastatic breast cancer.

Dr. McGovern also told me that after two-and-a-half years of chemotherapy he was taking me off of it and placing me instead on the maintenance drug Tamoxifen. He wanted me to understand that I had not failed chemo and that, if necessary, it would be reinstated at a future date. But, he explained, he wanted to wait a year to see what would transpire in my case. My blood was badly in need of some time off. "Most patients," he added, "can tolerate these powerful drugs for about a year, at best. You made it through thirty months—long enough to allow for the complete remission of a stage IV cancer, which is very rare indeed."

I suppose I should have been elated at the news of going off chemotherapy, but I wasn't. In fact, I was frightened by the idea. If these drugs had gotten me this far, I reasoned, why stop it now, especially since I had already tolerated its effects for this long? Now suddenly he's saying no more chemo? After he left the room, I just sat there wondering how long it would take before the cancer took its revenge. When I stepped into the hall, I could hardly walk. I remember leaning against the wall and softly weeping. I felt like a passenger in a boat that had been sailed far from shore and was now being told she had to jump out of the boat and swim back on her own.

After composing myself, I walked into the waiting room where Dick was sitting. I told him what the doctor had said. Like the good husband he is, he tried to be upbeat about it, saying that getting off of chemotherapy sounded like a good thing to him.

So, I was taken off the hard stuff and put on Tamoxifen, later replaced by Arimidex, which I have tolerated very well, with the exception of the occasional hot flash. Other than the infrequent infection at my catheter site, which led to its removal after three years, things went pretty smoothly for the next eighteen months. My fear of the worst had not become a reality. Four years after my original diagnosis, Dr. McGovern noted, “Patient continues to do well in state of complete remission.” Somehow, I had come back from the depths of stage IV adenocarcinoma and survived.

But my story was not over with yet.

XI

Eleven years would pass before the word malignancy came back into my life. During that interval, I had continued to take my Tamoxifen. I'd also continued to undergo my annual body scans, usually done in the fall of the year. These scans showed only a slowly progressive deterioration of bone in my back and ribs, as well as in most of my major joints. The culprit was not cancer but osteoporosis and arthritis, evidence (if any were needed) that I was aging.

As a cancer survivor who routinely took her maintenance medication for over a decade, it never occurred to me that I could develop the disease again. How wrong I was.

It started innocently enough. While chewing on a piece of peanut brittle one night in front of the TV in December of 2001, I happened to break off a piece of tooth. Because there was some pain involved, I made a dental appointment for the following week, expecting no more than a routine dental repair. Yet no sooner had I sat in the chair and opened my mouth than my dentist exclaimed, "My goodness, how long have you had that growing along the inside of your mouth? Certainly, it must be painful?" I didn't know what he was talking about. I had felt no oral pain that I could recall. The only symptom in fact that I'd experienced having to do with my mouth was a slight tenderness whenever my toothbrush bumped against the inside of my cheek, but that was it.

Because he was wary of the look of this suspicious patch of skin, my dentist decided to skip the tooth repair that day and instead sent me immediately down to Dr. McGovern's office for an oncological opinion. Well, Dr. McGovern didn't like the look of the inside of my cheek either and ordered a biopsy. When the lab report came back it read, "Biopsy of right tonsillar pillar reveals in situ, squamous cell carcinoma." I was told that 'in situ' meant that the cancer had not yet metastasized, or spread, beyond its original site. So, there was *some* good news anyway.

Although I had quit smoking after my original cancer diagnosis years ago, the effects of so many years of that bad habit had taken its toll. Dr. McGovern recommended an oral surgeon, Dr. James Clemens, another wonderful medical man, who resected (cut out) and lasered the cancerous patch of tissue lining the inside of my right cheek. It all happened so quickly in comparison to the four-year nightmare involving the stage IV adenocarcinoma, I was amazed. Here the cancer had been detected, biopsied, surgically removed, and the area healed, all in less than a month. The only ill effect of the entire process was that I could eat nothing but oatmeal for two weeks following the surgery, due to the pain. But once the involved area was fully healed, all felt well again. In addition, I had lost ten pounds in the bargain.

Dr. Clemens was not going to let go of me quite so easily, however, and for the next year I had to come to his office for a monthly examination. And I am very glad of it, because later that autumn he found a second patch of the same kind of suspicious tissue, this time at the base of my tongue, just inside my throat. A biopsy again revealed squamous cell carcinoma in situ, and again Dr. Clemens wasted no time in excising and lasering the area. Further examinations and tests afterward pointed toward a favorable prognosis, which has indeed been the case. I have been free of oral cancer for over fifteen years now.

But my naive notion that nothing could ever again compare with the terrifying ordeal of the inoperable carcinoma of fifteen years ago, was mistaken. Over the course of the next three years, I would undergo a series of physical upheavals that had only commenced with these twin bouts of oral cancer.

XII

Later that winter, on the last day of February, I was spending a quiet evening at home when I started to feel an uncomfortable pain in my chest. I had for years experienced angina and so thought little of the discomfort. But this time it didn't seem to be going away. When I mentioned this to Dick, he told me that I did look pale to him. In fact, too pale. He said he wanted me to go in and get checked, but I refused, explaining that I didn't feel that bad. Yet after a while I did start feeling worse. The pain was not only increasing in intensity, but the area affected—spreading over the center of my chest—had grown to about the size of a compact disc. I said that I was going to shower and if the pain had not subsided by then, I would go in and get checked. As I got undressed, however, I knew something was not right. For one thing, as a person who ordinarily perspired only from her head, I was surprised to find that my underclothing was soaked with perspiration. I was now also beginning to feel nauseated. After my shower, I told Dick to take me to the emergency room. It was just after midnight.

I had been foolish to wait so long before going in. Apparently, the warning signs of a heart attack for women are much more varied than that of men. The emergency room physician very quickly recognized that I was experiencing a coronary and immediately began the necessary procedures to prevent any more damage than had already occurred. Preliminary tests indicated that I had suffered what was called "an acute anterior myocardial infarction." I remember thinking of the irony that I, a stage IV breast cancer survivor, might actually die instead of a heart attack. Here, tonight. How ridiculous, I thought.

The cardiac specialist on call that night was Dr. Sarah Fenton, who quickly performed a catheterization, a procedure where they go in to view the extent of cardiac damage by feeding a catheter into the right femoral artery (through the leg) leading to the heart. But I gave them trouble. Not that I wanted to. It's just that I couldn't keep my legs from moving, whether from restlessness or whatever. I can recall being told fairly loudly that I *must* restrain myself from thrashing about. But, having been given several drugs, including morphine for pain, I seemed unable to follow the directions these good people were calling out. Poor Dr. Fenton. She told my family later that this constant movement alone could have brought fatal consequences. But fortunately, she persevered and the catheterization procedure was completed. Afterwards, she revealed to me that 80% of my cardiac muscle was no longer functioning, explaining that I had probably suffered a blockage of some kind, whether from a clot or a piece of free-floating plaque, they couldn't tell. In any case, the blockage had apparently resolved on its own. What she sent in a letter to my primary physician the following day was:

> Ventriculography shows that Yvonne had an extensive anterior infarction with an ejection fraction of 20-25%. Clinically, it appears that she most likely ruptured a plaque but that the thrombus resolved prior to catheterization. The patient still had R wave preservation at the time of presentation and this would give substantial hope that there may be some return of systolic function in the left anterior descending coronary artery distribution.

To the rest of us, Dr. Fenton explained that the good news was that although so much of my heart was presently nonfunctional, there was a fairly good chance the muscle tissue was only stunned and that I might be able to get back some of my heart function, perhaps 50% or more.

After ten days in intensive care, I was to undergo three months of physical therapy, with restrictions placed on me as to what I could and could not do for the time being, such as lifting or pushing things about. Once again, my family came to my aid, offering to help clean the house, cook meals, and the like. And of course, I still had Dick in my corner for support and assistance.

In the weeks that followed, I felt more easily tired and was often short of breath. Yet things slowly began to improve. The physical therapy, though not easy, was a great help. Soon I was swimming, as well as riding the stationary bike. I was in fact getting into the best shape I'd been in since I can't remember when. The plan was that after three months I would have a second echocardiogram to compare with the first in order to see how much, if any, of my heart muscle function had returned.

The follow-up echocardiogram, performed in May, surprisingly showed a significant return of myocardial function. In fact, Dr. Fenton, who was very much amazed by the results of the test, informed me that my heart was now functioning at 100%. Although she'd seen such a level of recovery before, she had never before known it to happen so quickly. After having suffered a major myocardial infarction only three months earlier, I was now being told by my cardiologist that it seemed as if I had never suffered a heart attack at all. My goodness, I thought, how fortunate could one person be?

I would find that out soon enough.

XIII

I was visiting my granddaughter in the hospital after she'd undergone breast reduction surgery and had mentioned offhandedly to the attending surgeon who was in the room at the time that I wished I could have had the procedure done myself when I was younger. My breasts have always been too large (it runs in the family) and, after so many years of my carrying around their extra weight, had given me lower back trouble for at least the past decade. Although my earlier breast cancer had originated in an area other than my breasts proper, the surgeon told me that their tissue would be among the most susceptible if the cancer ever returned. In addition, he said that with my history, a double mastectomy would be the better route to go. Besides, he reasoned, if their weight was giving me so much trouble, that was only one more reason I might benefit from their removal. I could hardly believe what I was hearing.

I mentioned the idea to my family doctor and he said he thought it was a good one. With these two opinions bolstering my courage, I went to Dr. McGovern and asked what he thought. He was not real keen on the idea, pointing out how well things had been going for me without a mastectomy. His basic concern was: why stir up possible trouble in an area that has proven stable? I told him I could see his point but that I would still like to have the procedure done if possible. He said he would recommend a surgeon if I really wanted to go ahead with it. Seeing his concern, as well as my husband's, who happened to agree with Dr. McGovern on this one, I told the doctor that I would go along with whatever the surgeon recommended.

The surgeon who was consulted said that the procedure should be done "without a doubt." And so it was. A routine biopsy of the mass of removed tissue showed calcification, among other minor age-related signs of deterioration, as well as a large amount of excess adipose tissue. At my age they had become dead weight and I was pleased to be rid of them. So was my lower back. Later I was fitted for a pair of breast/bra prostheses and have worn them ever since without a second thought. I now feel better and look better. Mission accomplished.

For several months after the surgery, though, I continued to notice an area on the right side of my chest which remained tender. I had hesitated seeing the doctor about the tenderness as I did not want to suddenly sound like a hypochondriac. Finally, however, because there was also some swelling in that area, I went to see my family physician who thought that the trouble was due to a bone spur growing on the end of a rib. He recommended I see a plastic surgeon to have it taken care of. But when the plastic surgeon saw me, he said without hesitation that he suspected it was a tumor. Oh lord, there was that word again. To make sure, the plastic surgeon ordered a chest scan to be added to the other routine scans and tests I was to undergo at my annual oncological review with Dr. McGovern coming up shortly.

As fortune would have it, all the tests came back negative, except for the added chest scan, which showed not only a suspicious mass in the tender area on the right side of my chest wall, but a second mass inside my right lung. Both would have to be biopsied. The mass along my chest wall turned out to be a harmless sack of fluid which drained as soon as the biopsy needle punctured it. The mass inside my lung, unfortunately, was not so harmless. Instead, the biopsy revealed a malignancy about the circumference of a quarter. It appeared that my old nemesis adenocarcinoma had returned after seventeen years.

Had that harmless sack of fluid not formed, prompting the added chest scan, the lung cancer would likely have gone undetected.

XIV

I went to see Dr. John Seccombe, the surgeon who would perform the operation to remove the tumor, during the last week of November. A soft-spoken man, he explained in detail how I would need to have the entire upper lobe of my right lung removed along with the tumor. He did have a few good things to add along the way, though, such as the fact that the procedure no longer required the cutting of any ribs, and that the muscles in the area would also be spared. He mentioned that as recently as three months ago they were still cutting ribs for the procedure, which entailed additional pain and a longer period of recovery for the patient. Now, he said, the operation involved only the spreading of ribs to get at the lung, thus allowing for a quicker recovery time and significantly less pain. He also mentioned how fortunate it was that the tumor was on the lateral side of the lung, as this meant there was less chance of the lymph nodes, which are located near the esophagus, testing positive for cancer. He would, he explained, be removing some dozen or more of these lymph nodes to be examined in the lab in order to be certain there was no metastasis involved. He also explained that he would have to remove much of the fatty tissue on my right side in order to get at the ribs. "I see," I said, surmising what I viewed as an opportunity, "I suppose you couldn't reach over while you're in there and do the left side at the same time?" He just smiled, indicating that the interview was over.

Before a person undergoes this type of surgery, the lungs are tested to determine the patient's breathing ability. This endeavor requires a person to hold their breath until they think they are going to pass out. And even though I ended up performing poorly on this test, Dr. Seccombe said that he could tell from simply talking to me that my lungs were in good enough condition to endure the stress of surgery.

The operation was set for November 30th. On that date Dick accompanied me to the hospital as usual. I have to say I was frightened to be going in for such a procedure. I'd never had cancer in a major organ before, even during that first awful bout with adenocarcinoma seventeen years earlier. Although at that time the cancer had spread to nearly every area of my body, it never invaded an organ. This time, however, the disease would claim much of my right lung. Yet I was glad that the tumor was at least operable this time around, something the first cancer hadn't been. In a matter of hours, I said to myself, I could be free of cancer once more. That's the thought I tried to keep in mind as they prepped me for surgery.

I remember one incident, though, which I think demonstrates the fearful state of mind I was in at the time. While I was being readied to be wheeled down to surgery, my family was asked to stand outside the door. Although the atmosphere for most of the morning had been very solemn, someone must have said something humorous out there, because I could hear the sounds of muted chuckles coming from the hall. Suddenly, all I could think of was that I was no longer a part of the healthy world going on outside my little room. Instead, I was lying in a hospital bed, and this time I'd be going under the knife. How strange that one can be surrounded by people and somehow still feel so utterly alone.

I don't recall much of the twenty-four hours following the operation, but my family tells me I sounded as if I were in a great deal of misery. Dr. Seccombe had warned that the surgery could leave a patient in pain for some time until the tissues had fully healed, and that even then there might be some lingering irritation in the area. Even so, I was informed that everything had gone smoothly and that the sixteen lymph nodes they removed with the lobe had all tested negative. I was indeed cancer-free once more. That news was worth any amount of pain and inconvenience to me —and I would definitely have my share of both before the lengthy process of healing was over.

After being released from the intensive care unit, I was placed in a regular hospital room for several more days of post-op care and observation. It was during this second phase of my stay that something unfortunate occurred. I was not responding to the pain medication they were giving me. Instead, I seemed to be in almost constant agony. This situation eventually led to my being hooked up to a morphine drip where I was given control of how often I would receive the pain medication. Every eight minutes I could push a button and receive a dose. Yet even this set up did not help control the kind of pain I was experiencing. I remember being in such bad shape that I began turning visitors away so they wouldn't have to see how awful I felt and looked.

Then one of my sons discovered something that explained a lot. While he was helping reposition me in my bed, he noticed that the area where I was lying was soaking wet. An investigation by the nursing staff, who up to this point were at a loss to explain my misery, led to the discovery that the morphine drip had not been properly hooked up. Turns out that the pain medication I thought I was pumping into my body was for the most part going directly into my mattress instead. For two days I had gone with practically no medication at all to relieve pain. By the time the nurses finally got me hooked up properly, however, I no longer cared, since by then the medication was working fine. To this day I am left to wonder how much it must have cost to keep my mattress doped up for all that time, during which I had continued to press that silly button every eight minutes.

When finally allowed to go home, I was still attached to a portable oxygen tank to assist my breathing. I would remain on oxygen for about a month, during which time I was instructed to keep up my breathing therapy. These exercises involved sucking in as hard as I could on a little hand-held plastic device in order to strengthen my lungs. After several weeks of this therapy, I was glad to finally be done with it.

The only real complication in the weeks following surgery was how much fluid my body was generating. The problem became such that I ended up having to return to the hospital three more times before it was brought under control. Two chest tubes were inserted on two separate occasions, from which they drained quarts of fluid at a time. During one surgical procedure for the problem, performed in the operating room, Dr. Seccombe drained 200cc from me. But still it kept accumulating.

By the third return visit, I vowed I wouldn't leave the hospital again until the problem was resolved. Dr. Seccombe, who had convened a group of specialists to brainstorm a solution, said he had never before encountered such a massive and consistent fluid accumulation and drainage. Not until December twenty-ninth, one month after the date of surgery, was I cleared to leave the hospital for good. But it would be months before I was fully healed. Yet that day of recovery did ultimately come, and today I can honestly say I feel wonderful, and that I'm very thankful for it.

A pleasant bonus was that post-operative chemotherapy was deemed unnecessary by Dr. McGovern. After eighteen years as my oncologist, he informed me during my final visit to his office that he was retiring as of June 1st. I mentioned to him how I once again felt like a person in a boat who has been brought far out from shore only to be told that she must now swim back on her own. "Yes," he said, smiling, "and you're still swimming." I can never thank him enough for all his years of professional care and concern.

Six months later I met with my new oncologist, Dr. Gerald Bayer, who wrote the following assessment of my oncological history in his notes:

1) Breast adenocarcinoma with skeletal metastasis in full remission.

2) Oral squamous cell carcinoma resected without evidence of recurrence.

3) Adenocarcinoma of the right lung resected with no evidence of recurrence by recent CT scan of chest.

I have often asked myself how any person could be fortunate enough to beat such odds time and again, but of course there is no answer to that. And although I have wondered at times how I can still be alive, in the end, all that matters, I guess, is that I am. Yet I'm no one special, and if I have made it through the difficult battlefield, taking each day only as it comes, even the bad ones, then anybody can, including you, whoever you are. It really does amount to not giving up on hope, or yourself, no matter what comes your way.

TIMELINE

FIRST YEAR:

Summer: Pain in upper right arm noticed. Continues to increase. Experiencing fatigue. Four separate exams over eight weeks reveal nothing out of the ordinary.

August 11: Bone scan performed.

August 12: Bone scan reveals advanced cancer along skeletal system, especially ribs, spinal column, pelvic area, and left femur.

August 12-22: Biopsies of resected tissue reveal adenocarcinoma, stage IV. Disease considered terminal. Numerous tests, X-rays, and scans follow. First chemotherapy treatment administered, a mixture of the cancer drugs Cytoxan, Methotrexate, & 5-FU.

August 24: First visit to oncology office after release from hospital. Receives second chemotherapy treatment.

September 21: Dr. McGovern notes, “Patient is experiencing severe depression, agitation, crying episodes, as well as marked fatigue due to chemo treatments.” Antidepressant Desyrel prescribed. Narcotic analgesic not tolerated well. Motrin & Tylenol 3 prescribed.

Late September: Pancytopenia (low blood counts) due to effects of chemo, causes shaking spell, vomiting. Hospitalized for transfusion.

October 19: Dr. McGovern notes, "Patient seems to be coming out of the woods. She is able to smile and laugh. A complete change in her overall appearance." Continues on anti-depressant. Taking only Motrin 800 mg for pain at this time.

November 16: Doctor notes, "Patient feeling basically very well. Pain almost totally resolved. Depression resolved with only occasional blue days. Responding extremely well to chemotherapy treatments. Little to no nausea or lack of appetite."

December 14: "Patient states she feels significantly better during the two weeks she is off treatment, as opposed to the two weeks immediately following chemo treatment. Hickman catheter implanted in chest for easier administration of chemotherapy."

<u>SECOND YEAR</u>:

March 7: "Patient is tolerating her chemotherapy very well without any significant ill effects. Cancer is currently in a

state of partial remission, as documented by recent bone scan."

April: Hospitalized for deep venous thrombophlebitis (lower leg blood clot). Anticoagulant Coumadin is prescribed.

May 16: Doctor notes, "Pain completely resolved. At this time her malignancy has no evidence of progressive symptomology."

May 31: Development of anemia due to chemotherapy. Transfusion ordered. Specific donor blood is requested and used.

June 13: Doctor notes, "I can detect no fullness in the axilla of right breast as previously described. Infection at site of Hickman catheter." Erythromycin 250 mg prescribed for infection.

August 1: White blood cell and platelet counts low again due to effects of chemotherapy. Chemo dose is reduced until problem resolves itself.

August 29: One-year anniversary of original diagnosis. Doctor notes, "Bone scan and chest X-ray show stabilization of her disease with no evidence of progression."

THIRD YEAR:

January 17: Doctor notes, "Bone scan done today was excellent."

March 13: Hospitalized again for low blood cell and platelet counts due to effect of chemotherapy. Chemo again reduced. Blood counts to be checked weekly for now.

April 10: Chemotherapy dosages continue to be reduced due to another episode of pancytopenia and its effects.

May 8: Doctor notes, "Patient's blood counts have tolerated her recent chemotherapy very well, therefore dosages will be increased to level intermediate between original and most recent doses."

June 5: Doctor notes, "Bone scan shows complete remission". Minor infection at catheter site. Antibiotics prescribed.

June 19: Edema noted in both legs and ankles. Recommendation to increase Maxide medication to daily dose.

August 28: Two-year anniversary of original diagnosis of stage IV carcinoma. Continues in clinical state of remission. Reduction of chemo doses due to low blood counts.

December 18: Doctor notes, "Patient still experiencing mild alopecia requiring wig."

<u>FOURTH YEAR</u>:

January 15: Doctor notes, "Patient continues to tolerate her chemotherapy well."

March 12: Doctor notes, "Bone scan today still shows <u>complete remission</u> of her disease. Patient continues to do exceptionally well. I am going to stop her chemotherapy and place her on Tamoxifen. She has not failed chemo and it may be reinstated at a future date if necessary."

May 14: Doctor notes, "Tolerating Tamoxifen well with only mild increase of hot flashes and weight gain. Mild edema noted."

October 29: Redness and pain around Hickman catheter site. Erythromycin prescribed. Doctor notes, "If catheter site continues to be a problem it will be pulled."

December 6: Hickman catheter removed. Doctor notes, "Patient's only complaint is hot flashes due to Tamoxifen therapy."

* * *

FIFTH YEAR:

September 14: Four years since original diagnosis. Dr. McGovern notes, "Patient continues to do well in state of complete remission."

TEN YEARS LATER:

Late December: Biopsy of right anterior tonsillar pillar (inside mouth) reveals multifocal in situ squamous cell carcinoma.

THE FOLLOWING YEAR:

January 15: Surgical resection and lasering of oral squamous cell carcinoma site.

Autumn: Second oral squamous cell carcinoma detected and resected. Prognosis good.

THIRD YEAR:

February 27: Suffers major myocardial infarction (heart attack). Eighty percent of heart muscle stunned into inactivity. Full recovery of heart function follows within three months. Is switched from Tamoxifen to Arimidex because of its low thrombotic (clot-inducing) potential.

November 3: Doctor notes, "Patient continues to tolerate Arimidex well."

FOURTH YEAR:

Summer: Doctor notes, "Double mastectomy performed at patient's request. Area of hemorrhage and/or necrosis of the right surgical incision proves problematic."

November 16: Doctor notes, "Over several preceding months patient has developed cough and some new nodules on her chest wall where she has had mastectomies. Has suspicious mass on chest wall reminiscent of malignancy, possibly fat necrosis."

November 21: Chest scan reveals second mass in upper lobe of right lung.

November 23: Biopsy of mass on right wall benign. Biopsy of right lung lesion reveals adenocarcinoma.

Late November: Surgical removal of upper lobe of right lung containing "non-small cell adenocarcinoma." No lymph node involvement detected. Prognosis good. Chemotherapy deemed unnecessary.

FIFTH YEAR:

June 1: Retirement of Dr. James McGovern after eighteen years as oncologist.

August 18: Assessment of cancer history by new oncologist, Dr. Gerald Bayer:

1) Breast adenocarcinoma with skeletal metastasis still in full remission.

2) Oral squamous cell carcinomas in situ resected and lasered without evidence of recurrence.

3) Adenocarcinoma of right lung resected with no evidence of recurrence.

* * *

On August 8, 2014, after a further decade of cancer-free life, Yvonne Marie Pigeon dies at the age of 80, surviving her husband, Dick, by six years.

Made in United States
North Haven, CT
05 November 2026

21785837R00049